CANCER AND MODERN SCIENCE™

THYROID CANCER

Current and Emerging Trends in Detection and Treatment

JERI FREEDMAN

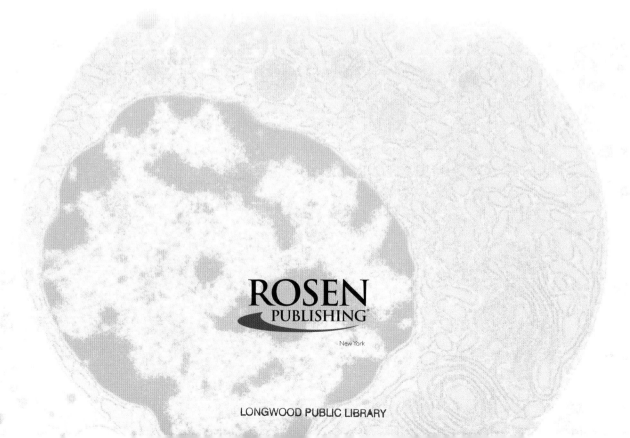

ROSEN
PUBLISHING®

New York

Published in 2012 by The Rosen Publishing Group, Inc.
29 East 21st Street, New York, NY 10010

Library of Congress Cataloging-in-Publication Data

Freedman, Jeri.
Thyroid cancer: current and emerging trends in detection and treatment / Jeri
Freedman.—1st ed.
     p. cm.—(Cancer and modern science)
Includes bibliographical references and index.
ISBN 978-1-4488-1308-7 (library binding)
1. Thyroid gland—Cancer. I. Title.
RC280.T6F74 2012
616.99'444—dc22

                                                          2010007710

Manufactured in the United States of America

CPSIA Compliance Information: Batch #S11YA: For further information, contact Rosen Publishing, New York, New York, at 1-800-237-9932.

On the cover: This photograph, taken through an electron microscope, shows a thyroid cancer cell. The nucleus *(center)* of the cell is abnormally large because cancer cells are abnormally active.

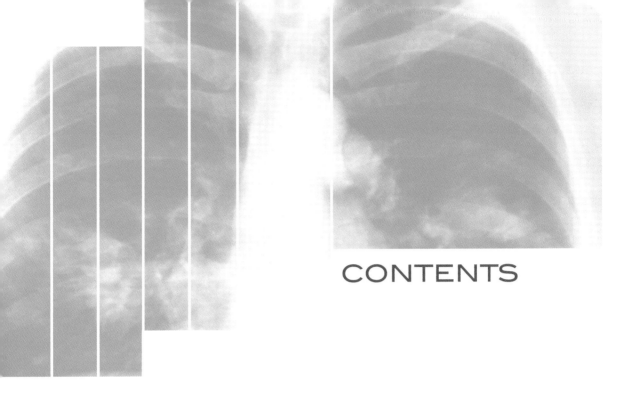

CONTENTS

INTRODUCTION

The thyroid gland is a butterfly-shaped organ located in the front of the throat below the Adam's apple. A gland is an organ that produces a type of chemical compound called a hormone. Hormones leave glands through an opening called a duct. They travel through the bloodstream to other organs in the body and regulate their functioning. There are many types of glands and hormones in the body. The thyroid gland is one of the most important because the hormones that it produces affect the entire body's metabolism (chemical processes that occur in the body). It influences the body's reaction to other hormones and its utilization of energy, among other processes. The thyroid gland is part of a larger system of glands called the endocrine system.

Knowledge of the thyroid gland and thyroid diseases dates back to the end of the nineteenth century. The man who first discovered the function of the thyroid gland was a Swiss surgeon named Theodor Kocher (1841–1917). Kocher was the first surgeon to remove the thyroid gland to treat thyroid disease. His observation of the effects of this

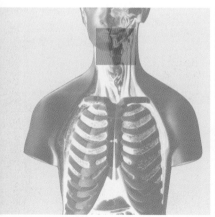 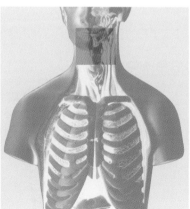 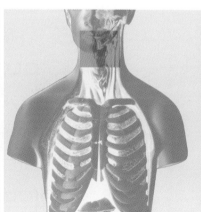

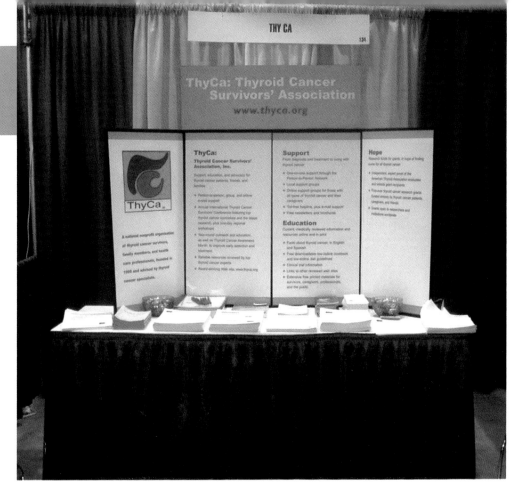

The Thyroid Cancer Survivors' Association reaches out to the public, patients, caregivers, and health care professionals to provide free support services and education about all types of thyroid cancer.

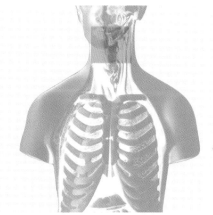

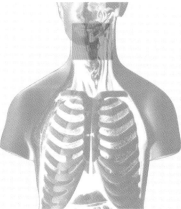

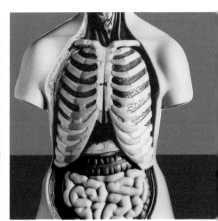

surgery on the patient's body was key to understanding the functions that thyroid hormones perform in the body.

Thyroid cancer is the uncontrolled growth of thyroid cells, which form lumps called nodules and disrupt the functioning of the thyroid gland. Thyroid cancer is relatively rare, accounting for only about 1 percent of all cancers. Unlike many other types of cancer, thyroid cancer is usually treatable and rarely fatal. Since the late 1990s, the incidence of thyroid cancer has been rising about 8 percent annually. However, according to the National Cancer Institute and a number of independent studies, a significant portion of the increase is most likely the result of improved detection methods.

Even though thyroid cancer is usually treatable, it is a serious disease. Getting appropriate treatment right away is important. This book begins by discussing how the thyroid functions. It then examines what thyroid cancer is and how it is diagnosed and treated. It goes on to look at what recovery from treatment is like and what kind of follow-up can be expected. Finally, it discusses current research that might lead to new methods of diagnosis and treatment for thyroid cancer.

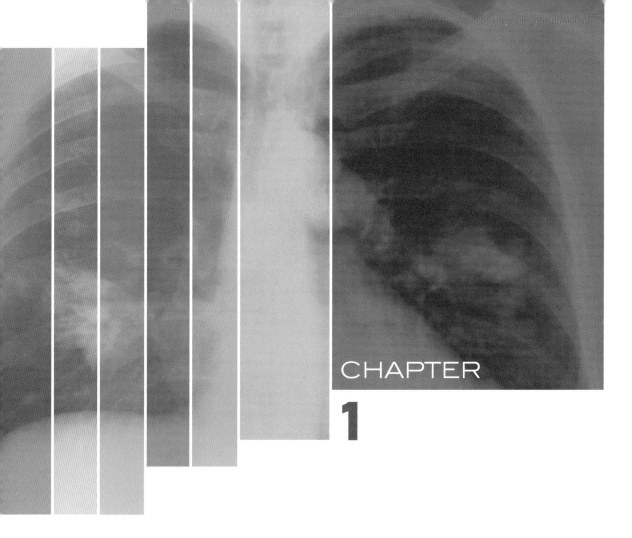

WHAT IS THYROID CANCER?

The thyroid gland is composed of two segments called lobes, which contain spherical pouches called follicles. The follicles absorb iodine from the diet. The thyroid gland uses this iodine to produce its hormones. Most of the iodine consumed today comes from table salt. Other good sources are seafood and dairy products.

A layer of epithelial cells surrounds the follicles. Epithelial cells are those that cover or line a gland or organ. The epithelial thyroid cells secrete (release) the thyroid hormones thyroxine (T4) and tri-iodothyronine (T3), which pass into the bloodstream. In the spaces

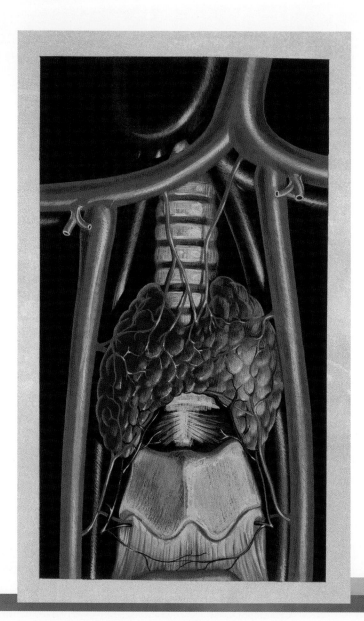

This illustration shows the location of the thyroid gland in the throat. It sits on top of the cartilage in the throat, making it easy to feel any abnormal growths.

between the follicles are parafollicular cells, called C cells. These cells produce the hormone calcitonin, which helps regulate calcium usage in the body.

Thyroid Hormones

Thyroid hormones are produced in a feedback loop, a process in which the amount of the hormone that starts the process is increased or decreased according to the level of the final product in the blood. The cycle doesn't start in the thyroid gland but in an organ in the center of the brain called the hypothalamus. The hypothalamus produces thyroid-releasing hormone (TRH). TRH stimulates a small gland at the base of the brain called the pituitary gland. TRH causes this gland to produce thyroid-stimulating hormone (TSH), which then travels to the thyroid gland. When TSH reaches the thyroid gland, it stimulates it to start producing the thyroid hormones T4 and T3, which attach to blood proteins produced by the liver. They travel through the bloodstream to tissues located throughout the body and attach to receptors on cells that are all over the body. They control the rate at which cells use oxygen and energy from food. If the levels of thyroid hormones in the body are not correct, the body's organs will not function properly.

The body contains chemical sensors that monitor its levels of hormones. As the levels of T3 and T4 rise, these sensors signal to the hypothalamus, which reduces the amount of TRH it makes. The reduction in TRH then causes the pituitary gland to decrease production of TSH, which then results in less T3 and T4 being produced by the thyroid. As the levels of T3 and T4 drop, the reverse process takes place: The hypothalamus puts out more TRH, the pituitary gland increases the output of TSH, and the thyroid gland puts out more T3 and T4. In this way, the levels of thyroid hormones, and thus the body's metabolism, remain optimal.

PIONEERING THYROID TREATMENT

Emil Theodor Kocher (1841–1917) was born in Bern, Switzerland, and studied medicine in Zurich, Berlin, London, and Vienna. In 1872, he became professor of surgery and director of the surgical clinic in Bern. At the time that Kocher was practicing medicine, goiter (enlarged thyroid) was a major problem in Bern because of the lack of iodine in the diet of the inhabitants. Kocher pioneered partial and full removal of the thyroid to treat goiter. However, in following his patients after their thyroids had been removed, he observed that many people developed the mental and physical symptoms of hypothyroidism. These symptoms included weight gain, excessive tiredness, and frequently feeling cold. What Kocher learned enabled him to improve the approach to thyroid removal. He wrote a book titled *Erkrankungen der Schilddrüse* (*Diseases of the Thyroid Gland*), which describes the symptoms and course of thyroid disease and the treatment of goiters. In 1909, Kocher was awarded the Nobel Prize for his work on thyroid surgery. He used his Nobel Prize money to fund the Kocher Clinic in Bern.

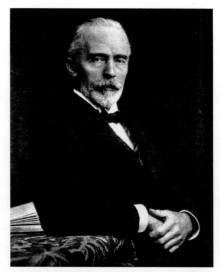

Emil Theodor Kocher pioneered surgery for treatment of thyroid disease. He also developed a number of surgical instruments.

Unfortunately, many things can go wrong in this complex system, leading to too much or too little T3 and T4 being produced. When too little of these thyroid hormones is produced, the condition is called hypothyroidism; when too much is produced, the condition is called hyperthyroidism.

What Is Thyroid Cancer?

Cancer occurs when cells grow out of control, forming large masses of malfunctioning cells that can damage surrounding tissue and interfere with the functioning of organs. Thyroid nodules can be considered benign or malignant. "Malignant" means cancer cells can spread to other parts of the body. This process is called metastasis. "Benign" means not cancerous, although benign tumors can cause problems because they take up space within vital organs and can affect their function. Although people of all ages can get benign nodules, they are most common in older people. Only about 5 percent of nodules found in the thyroid are cancerous.

How Thyroid Cancer Affects the Body

According to the American Cancer Society, thyroid cancer is the least fatal type of cancer. Five-year survival is an important measure of how successful medical care is in treating cancer. Ninety-seven percent of people who develop thyroid cancer are still alive five years later. Although it is rarely fatal if treated promptly and properly, thyroid cancer has a number of effects on the body.

A small number of nodules in the thyroid gland may produce few symptoms, but a large number of nodules or large nodules themselves may affect the gland's ability to produce the correct amount of thyroid hormone. Producing too much thyroid hormone, or hyperthyroidism, causes nervousness, excessive hunger, weight loss,

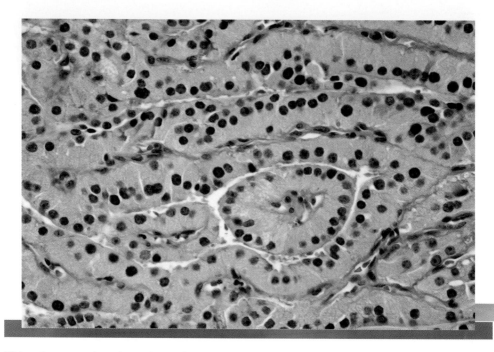

This photograph, taken through a microscope, shows Hürthle cell cancer of the thyroid gland. The cells in this type of tumor have very small uniform nuclei.

sleeplessness, a feeling of being too warm, and an irregular heart-beat. Having too little thyroid hormone is called hypothyroidism. Hypothyroidism causes weight gain, fatigue (lack of energy), and sensitivity to cold.

In addition to thyroid hormone–related problems, the nodules that form in the neck can put pressure on other structures in the neck, such as the lymph nodes and parathyroid glands, which are located on the underside of the thyroid. Damage to the parathyroid glands can cause a variety of problems in the body by disrupting calcium levels, which are controlled in part by the parathyroid glands. In some cases, nodules may get large enough to press on the esophagus (the tube in the throat con-

THYROID CANCER STATISTICS

According to the American Cancer Society:

— In 2009, there were about thirty-seven thousand cases of thyroid cancer in the United States. About three-quarters of those cases occurred in women.

— About 1,600 people died of thyroid cancer in 2009.

— Close to two-thirds of thyroid cancer occurs in people between the ages of twenty and fifty-five.

— According to Statistics Canada: thyroid cancer is the most common form of cancer in people who are ages twenty to thirty-nine.

necting the mouth to the stomach) or the trachea (windpipe). If a nodule presses on the esophagus, a person can have difficulty swallowing. If it presses on the trachea, it may cause breathing problems. When nodules become that big, it is necessary to remove them, regardless of whether they are malignant or benign.

The next chapter explains how cancer occurs and the different types of thyroid cancer.

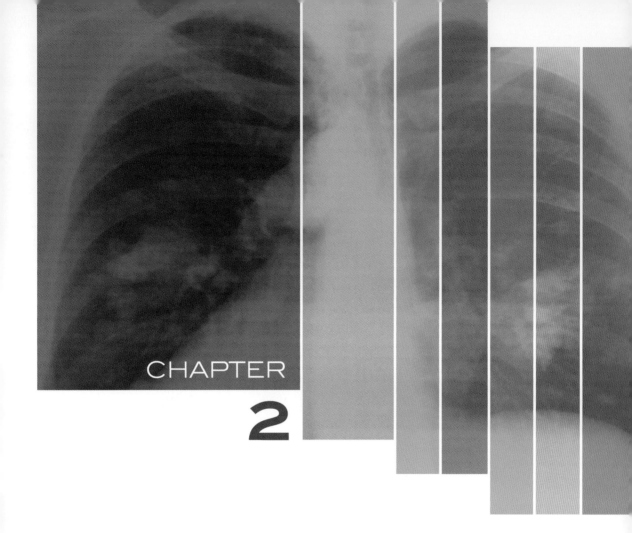

THE SCIENCE OF THYROID CANCER

Cancer occurs when cells grow out of control. What causes the cells to grow uncontrollably? Most cells in the human body reproduce numerous times over the course of a person's life. Every time a cell reproduces, its genetic material—in the form of units called genes—is copied. In this copying process, small errors, called mutations, often occur. Most of these mutations have no effect on how the cell functions because the body recognizes its mistakes and quickly fixes or gets rid of them. However, it is possible for the mistakes to affect the part of the

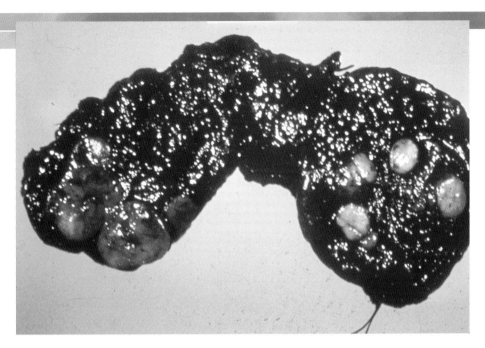

This thyroid gland is filled with cancerous nodules. The nodules can be felt in the gland by touch. Being fast-growing thyroid gland cells, they secrete abnormal amounts of thyroid hormones.

gene that turns cellular reproduction on or off. If a change leads to a gene for growth being turned on, the cell can keep reproducing uncontrollably, leading to the development of a tumor. The same thing can happen if a change damages a gene that turns off reproduction. When the cells grow out of control, they invade tissues in the body, causing damage to organs. If cancer is not treated, some cells can break off from the cluster and travel through the bloodstream to other organs. There, the cells continue to reproduce, invading the tissue nearby and damaging that organ. This process by which cancer cells spread from one organ to another is called metastasis.

THE TYPES OF THYROID CANCER

Various types of thyroid cancer affect different cells found in the thyroid. There are several types of thyroid cancer, including papillary, follicular, medullary, and anaplastic. It is important to identify the type of thyroid cancer a person has because the kind affects which treatment is most likely to work and how successful the treatment will likely be. The most common types of thyroid cancer are papillary and follicular. These types of tumors are slower growing and rarely fatal. The faster-growing and more primitive type is called anaplastic thyroid cancer, which is harder to treat. The following sections describe the various types of thyroid cancer.

PAPILLARY AND FOLLICULAR CANCERS

There are several types of thyroid cancer that arise from specific cells within the thyroid: papillary, follicular, and Hürthle cell. These three types all come from follicular cells that are growing out of control and are called carcinomas (cancers). Papillary carcinoma is the most common type. It is usually slow growing and tends to occur in only one lobe of the thyroid gland, although it can occur in both lobes. Papillary carcinomas tend to have a good outcome with prompt treatment. Sometimes these cancers spread to the lymph nodes in the neck. Lymph nodes produce fluid containing immune system cells to fight infection. Even when it spreads to the lymph nodes, papillary carcinoma can usually be treated successfully.

Follicular cancer, also called follicular adenocarcinoma, is the second most common type of thyroid cancer. About 10 percent of thyroid cancer cases are the follicular subtype. Although follicular cancer does not usually spread to the lymph nodes in the neck, it can spread to other locations, including the lungs and bones. It is more difficult to treat than

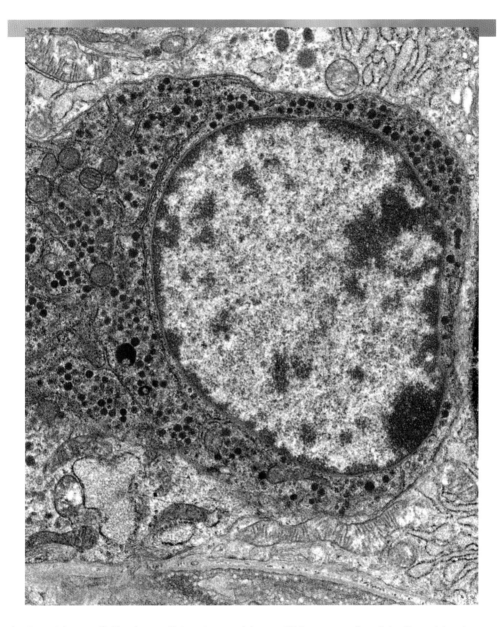

A thyroid parafollicular cell is pictured here. This type of cell is found in the connective tissue located adjacent to the thyroid follicles.

papillary cancer, but the chances of success are still high. Follicular cancer mostly occurs in people over the age of fifty. It is not uncommon to also encounter a mixed papillary-follicular cancer, which contains both types of cancer cells. This type of cancer is also highly treatable.

OTHER THYROID CANCERS

In addition to differentiated follicular cancers, there are several other thyroid cancers. These are rare and generally account for a small percentage of thyroid cancers. Medullary thyroid cancer (MTC) develops from the C cells in the thyroid. It represents about 5 percent of thyroid cancers. Because this type of cancer comes from C cells, it secretes calcitonin. It also secretes a protein called carcinoembryonic antigen, which is produced by other types of cancers as well. Both compounds can be detected by a blood test. Unfortunately, this type of cancer metastasizes easily and often spreads to the liver, lungs, or lymph nodes before a nodule is large enough to be noticed. Because it doesn't easily absorb radioactive iodine, it is more difficult to treat than many other types of thyroid cancer.

About 20 percent of MTC is hereditary and occurs as part of genetic syndromes. This type of MTC can occur in children or young adults. Hereditary MTC often occurs in both lobes of the thyroid, and people who have it may have other types of tumors as well. Eighty percent of MTC cases are not linked to genetics, though. This type of MTC is called sporadic MTC because it occurs occasionally and unpredictably.

Another rare type of thyroid cancer is anaplastic carcinoma. It accounts for only 2 percent of thyroid cancers. This is an undifferentiated type of thyroid cancer, which means the cells do not look like clearly developed thyroid cells under the microscope. Anaplastic carcinoma is very aggressive and spreads rapidly. It is difficult to treat and mostly occurs in people over the age of sixty.

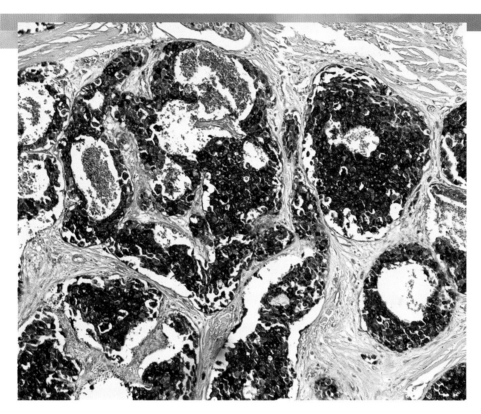

A fourteen-year-old's cancerous medullary cells in the thyroid gland are seen in this photograph. Cells from this type of tumor spread easily to other organs in the body.

Another very rare cancer occurring in the thyroid is lymphoma, which is not a true thyroid cancer but a cancer of the immune system cells found in lymph nodes, such as those in the neck. It mostly occurs in people over seventy years old.

RISK FACTORS
There are a number of different types of risk factors for thyroid cancer. Some factors are environmental, some are genetic, and some relate to

other medical conditions. The following sections provide the details on all these risk factors.

RADIATION

From the 1940s through the 1960s, low-dose radiation treatments were used to treat problems such as birthmarks on the neck and lower face, acne, and tonsillitis. Having had this treatment can make one more likely to develop thyroid cancer. Having had radiation treatment for another type of cancer, Hodgkin's lymphoma, can also increase one's chances of getting thyroid cancer. Hodgkin's lymphoma affects the lymph nodes, so radiation is sometimes used in the region of the neck.

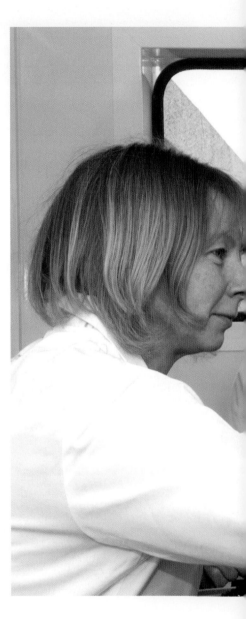

Having had radiation treatment increases one's risk of thyroid cancer because radiation can damage cells' genes, producing mutations that result in uncontrolled growth of damaged cells when those cells reproduce. Exposure to radiation from other sources can also put one at risk for thyroid cancer. For instance, radiation from nuclear bomb testing or nuclear power plant accidents can put one at risk. For that reason, people living within

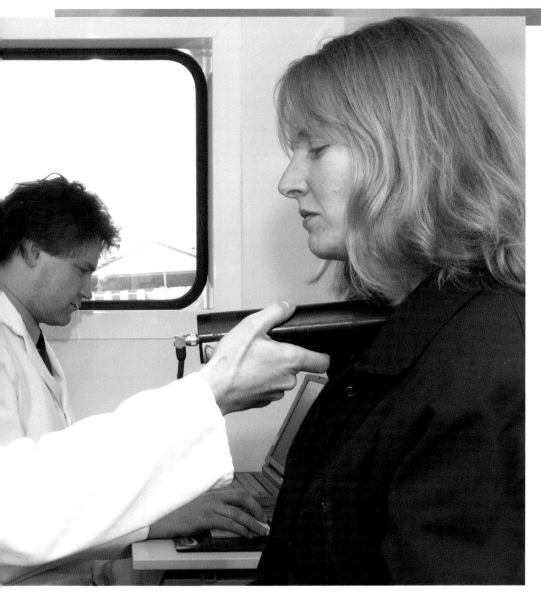

A scientist uses a probe to measure the amount of radioactive iodine present in a patient's thyroid gland. The sodium iodide crystal lights up when radiation reacts with it.

10 miles (16 kilometers) of a nuclear power plant may be eligible to receive potassium iodide pills to keep on hand in case there is a radiation leak from the power plant. This medication keeps radiation from affecting the thyroid.

CHERNOBYL AND RESEARCH INTO THYROID CANCER

In 1986, a nuclear reactor at a power plant in the city of Chernobyl in Ukraine on the border of Belarus exploded, exposing people who lived in the area around the plant to high levels of radiation. This tragic event resulted in the inhabitants developing many different types of cancer, including thyroid cancer. Numerous studies have recorded a significantly higher incidence of thyroid cancer among those exposed to the radiation. This is particularly notable in children who were exposed because the thyroid in children is more sensitive to radiation. Between 1986 and 1995 more than five hundred cases of thyroid cancer were found in people exposed to the radiation as children. Studies indicate that as many as 30 percent of children exposed to radiation develop thyroid cancer. Researchers are continuing to study the survivors of the Chernobyl disaster to learn about the effects of exposure to high levels of radiation on cancer. To support this effort, an international effort has been undertaken to establish a tissue and data bank with information from those affected by the Chernobyl disaster for study. Involved in the effort are the governments of Belarus, the Russian Federation, and Ukraine; the National Cancer Institute of the United States; the European Commission; the Saskawa Memorial Health Foundation of Japan; and the World Health Organization.

GENETICS

Genetics can play a role in certain types of thyroid cancer, such as medullary thyroid cancer. If a person has a defect in a gene that leads him or her to develop thyroid cancer, it is possible for that defective gene to be passed down to the person's descendants. When that happens, the person who inherits the defective gene has a higher likelihood of getting thyroid cancer. The gene linked to medullary thyroid cancer is called the RET oncogene ("onco" is a prefix meaning "cancer"). The gene can be detected by genetic testing. If thyroid cancer runs in a person's family, he or she may want to consult a genetic counselor. This person can provide information about genetic testing and the pros and cons. Some people who know they have the RET oncogene choose to have their thyroid gland removed to eliminate the chance of developing thyroid cancer. It is important to note that not everyone who inherits a defective gene will get cancer, though. Often, more than one negative factor is necessary to induce cancer.

AGE

Age is another factor that affects the likelihood of a person getting thyroid cancer. The older a person is, the more likely he or she is to develop all types of cancer, including thyroid cancer. After age seventy, people are especially vulnerable to this complication because of the number of times the cells have reproduced. The more times a cell is copied, the more likely it is that a damaging change will occur and that more changes will accumulate. Since the older a person is, the more times his or her cells have been copied, the more likely it is that a tumor-producing mutation will occur in an older person.

MYTHS AND FACTS

MYTH If my thyroid is enlarged, that means I have thyroid cancer.

FACT A swollen thyroid, called a goiter, is most often the result of other types of thyroid disease or too little iodine in the diet. There are many diseases that cause thyroid swelling that are not cancer. Thyroid cancer is actually quite rare, especially in children and teens.

MYTH Teenagers don't get thyroid cancer.

FACT Thyroid cancer does occur in children and teenagers, especially if they have been exposed to radiation for medical treatment or from the environment, or if they have a hereditary form of the disease.

MYTH Iodized table salt is unnatural and, therefore, unhealthy. Consequently, one should stick to natural forms, like sea salt.

FACT A lack of dietary iodine is a risk factor for thyroid cancer. Adding iodine to table salt has radically reduced the occurrence of thyroid problems because it is difficult to get enough dietary iodine, especially in areas where little iodine occurs in the soil.

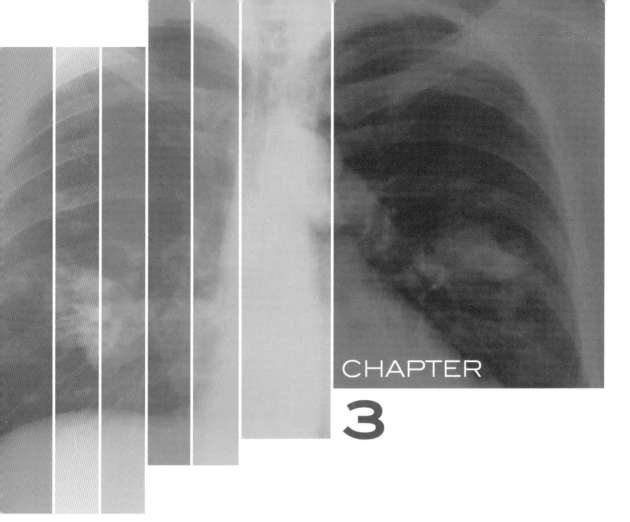

DETECTION AND TREATMENT

Detecting thyroid cancer is not always easy because the symptoms of thyroid problems can mimic those of other diseases. In addition, the symptoms of thyroid cancer can resemble those of other thyroid problems. Because thyroid cancer is rare, the examining doctor may initially assume that the problem is a more common thyroid problem. There are tests that can help distinguish thyroid cancer from other problems, though. Some of these tests are noninvasive and can be done without penetrating the body. Others require directly sampling blood or tissue.

Symptoms of Thyroid Cancer

According to the Mayo Clinic, an organization that provides clinic and hospital services and is based in Rochester, Minnesota, the symptoms of thyroid cancer include the following:

— A lump that can be felt in the neck
— Pain in the neck
— Difficulty swallowing
— Hoarseness
— A persistent cough that is not related to infection
— Swelling in the lymph nodes

Problems with the thyroid are often more difficult to diagnose in elderly people than in younger people because they often have other ailments that produce similar symptoms.

How Thyroid Cancer Is Diagnosed

Because of its location at the front of the throat, the thyroid gland is easy to see and feel. Often, patients or doctors can touch the thyroid gland and feel that it is bigger than usual or it contains bumps. Enlargement of the thyroid is called goiter. Although it may be present when a person has thyroid cancer, it can be caused by other conditions as well. For instance, if a person has a deficiency (reduced amount) of thyroid hormone in his or her body because of a lack of iodine in the diet, the thyroid may swell and become enlarged because it is working harder to try to produce more of the hormone. As mentioned earlier, many nodules in the thyroid are noncancerous. Most of these are cysts filled with colloid. However, some are solid, and this type includes hyperplastic nodules and adenomas. Although these solid types are not considered

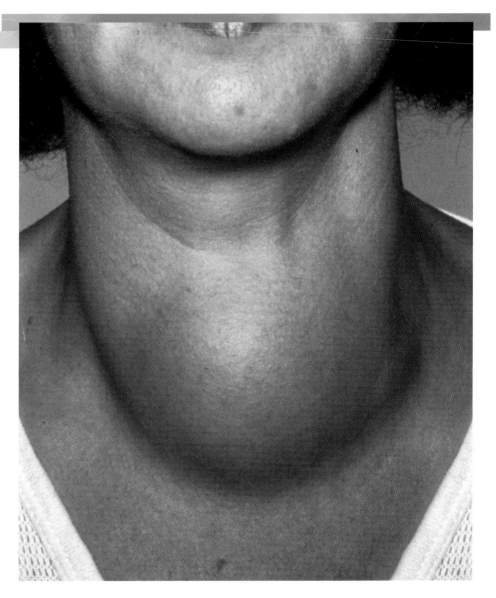

This person has a goiter, a swollen thyroid gland. Goiters result when the thyroid gland does not receive enough iodine in the diet to efficiently produce thyroid hormones.

cancerous, they can secrete excess thyroid hormone, which can cause symptoms of hyperthyroidism. In that case, the nodules may need to be treated or removed, even though they are not cancer.

The doctor may also use a laryngoscope to examine the thyroid. A laryngoscope is a flexible tube that the doctor inserts into the patient's throat. It has a tiny light and video camera on it that allow the doctor to view the structures in the throat on a monitor. If a doctor suspects that a person has a thyroid disorder, he or she may order blood tests. A blood test will show if the levels of thyroid hormones in the body are normal. If there is too much or too little, this indicates a thyroid problem.

IMAGING

Imaging scans are also used to examine the thyroid directly. The most commonly used initial imaging test for thyroid cancer is ultrasound. In an ultrasound test, a technician moves a handheld device over the patient's neck. The device bounces sound waves off the thyroid and surrounding structures. The signals coming back are transmitted to a computer, which analyzes them and produces an image of the structures on a monitor. Medical professionals can directly view anything abnormal, such as nodules, in this way. Thyroid ultrasound has improved the detection of thyroid cancer by detecting nodules too small to be noticed by other means. If the doctor suspects that cancer may be present, he or she will most likely order a biopsy.

BIOPSY

A biopsy is a test in which a small piece of tissue is removed and examined under a microscope to see if cancerous cells are present. If the biopsy indicates that there are cancer cells in the thyroid, the doctor may order a radionuclide scan of the patient's body. In a radionuclide scan, the patient is given a dose of mildly radioactive iodine. The iodine is taken up by thyroid cells, including cancerous ones that have spread to other parts of the body. A special camera called a radionuclide scanner is moved over the body. It produces an image of each part of the body examined. It detects radiation, so any thyroid cancer cells that have spread to organs other than the thyroid show up on the scan. This allows the doctor to know whether or not the cancer has spread and, if so, where it has spread.

THE STAGES OF THYROID CANCER

After the examination and testing take place, the resulting information is used in a process called staging the cancer. This process describes how severe the cancer is, based on the following details:

— Where the cancer is located
— Whether or not it has spread to other organs, and if so, which ones
— Whether or not it has spread to the lymph nodes
— What type of cancer cell is involved

These elements affect what types of treatment are used to treat the cancer and the likelihood of treating it successfully. A standard method that is often used for staging cancer is the TNM system. In this system, the T represents the size of the tumor, the N stands for whether the lymph nodes are involved, and the M stands for metastasis. The severity of cancer is also classified according to four stages. In the case of thyroid cancer, the stages are as follows:

— Stage 1: The cancer is confined to the thyroid.
— Stage 2: The cancer is a larger tumor, there are several tumors within the thyroid, or the cancer has spread to structures adjacent to the thyroid gland.

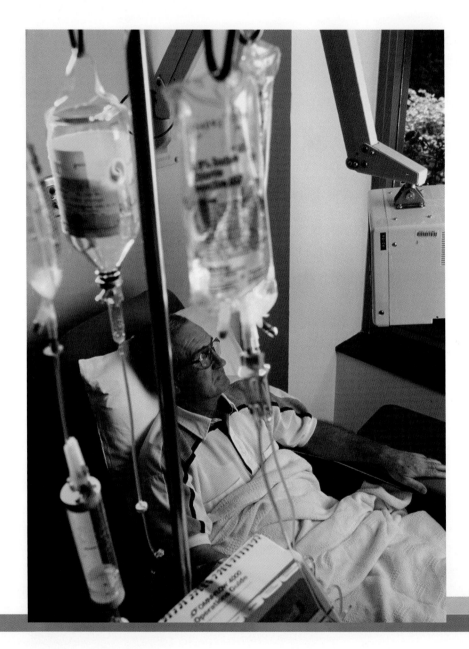

This patient is undergoing chemotherapy for cancer. In chemotherapy, strong chemicals are used to kill fast-growing cells, including cancer cells.

— Stage 3: The cancer has spread to the lymph nodes.
— Stage 4: The cancer has metastasized.

In cases where the thyroid cancer has recurred, which means the cancer has come back after treatment, doctors may give a new stage to the cancer. The new stage is based on how far the cancer has spread. According to the American Cancer Society, this staging is not typically as formal a process as the first cancer staging.

TREATMENTS FOR THYROID CANCER

Treatment for thyroid cancer usually involves surgery. The surgery for thyroid cancer consists of removal of the thyroid gland through an incision (cut) in the neck. Sometimes only one lobe is removed, but more commonly the entire thyroid gland is removed. This procedure is called a thyroidectomy. Sometimes the lymph nodes are removed, too. The lymph nodes will be checked under a microscope to see if the cancer has spread from the thyroid to the lymphatic system. Sometimes a small amount of thyroid tissue is left in place to protect the parathyroid glands.

A thyroidectomy is frequently followed by treatment with radioactive iodine to kill any stray cancer cells. It is also used to kill cancer cells that have spread to other parts of the body. The iodine is given to the patient in either liquid or pill form. The iodine travels through the bloodstream. Because thyroid cells readily absorb iodine, the radioactive iodine is taken up by the cancerous thyroid cells wherever they have lodged in the body. The radiation kills the cancer cells. Some patients may stay in the hospital for a few days during treatment in a special lead-lined room to prevent the radiation from affecting others. The type of radioactive material used only lasts for a short time and is excreted from the body in urine. There are some initial side effects from the treatment, which may include nausea, dry mouth and eyes, and pain in the location where cancer cells are being killed. During treatment, patients have to be careful not to expose other people to the radiation in their body, especially children and pregnant women.

There are a couple of less commonly used treatments that are sometimes employed in treating thyroid cancer, especially in cases that are harder to treat with radioactive iodine. The first is external radiation therapy. In this type of treatment, the patient lies on a table while a machine delivers a concentrated dose of radiation to carefully targeted sites on his or her body. This treatment is administered a few minutes at a time over a number of weeks. A second approach is chemotherapy. In this approach, the patient is given strong chemicals that kill fast-growing cells, including cancer cells. This treatment is usually given in several doses over a number of months. Both external radiation and chemotherapy have a number of side effects, including nausea, fatigue, and temporary hair loss.

WHAT IS RADIOACTIVE IODINE?

All elements are made up of atoms. An atom has protons and neutrons at its center, the nucleus. Protons have a positive electrical charge, whereas neutrons are neutral. Surrounding the nucleus are an equal number of electrons, which have a negative electrical charge. Radioactive iodine is also called iodine-131. Ordinary iodine is called iodine-127 because an atom of iodine has 127 protons and neutrons in its nucleus. Iodine-131 has the same number of protons as iodine-127, but it has 131 neutrons. This difference makes iodine-131 unstable, so it interacts with the atoms in tissue. Iodine-131 is one of the products produced by splitting atoms of uranium. Iodine-131 does not last long in the body. The younger a person is, however, the faster it clears from the body.

Alternative and Complementary Treatments

In addition to medical treatment, there are a variety of complementary activities that some patients find useful when dealing with cancer. These techniques are called complementary for a reason. They may be a helpful addition to treatment, but they are not a substitute for conventional medical treatment. Still, in some cases, they can help ease the symptoms of the disease or the side effects and stress of treatment.

Acupuncture is a traditional Chinese art that some people find helps with pain and nausea from radiation and chemotherapy treatments. In acupuncture, a practitioner inserts thin needles at key points around the body. When properly placed, the needles are thought to affect organs distant from the point of insertion. Massage therapy is another way of helping a person relax and reducing stress. In massage therapy, a massage therapist manipulates muscles to relax them. When a person has cancer, muscle spasms (tightening of the muscles) can occur as a result of the treatment or from stress. Therapeutic massage can relieve muscle spasms, thereby reducing pain.

The theory behind imagery techniques is that they can be used to focus the mind so that it influences the body to fight the cancer. There are various approaches to imagery. In one form, patients picture themselves in a pleasant situation, such as lying on a beach, in order to relax. In another type of imaging, patients picture the cancer being destroyed. Although imagery techniques don't cure cancer, they can help patients by inducing relaxation and reducing stress. In addition, concentrating one's mind on improving the state of one's health can influence one to do things that make the body better able to heal, such as eating better. A more formal approach to calming the mind and body is meditation. In meditation, the practitioner follows a series of procedures, such as breathing in a certain way, which stills his or her thoughts and/or focuses the mind. Meditation can relax the body and reduce stress.

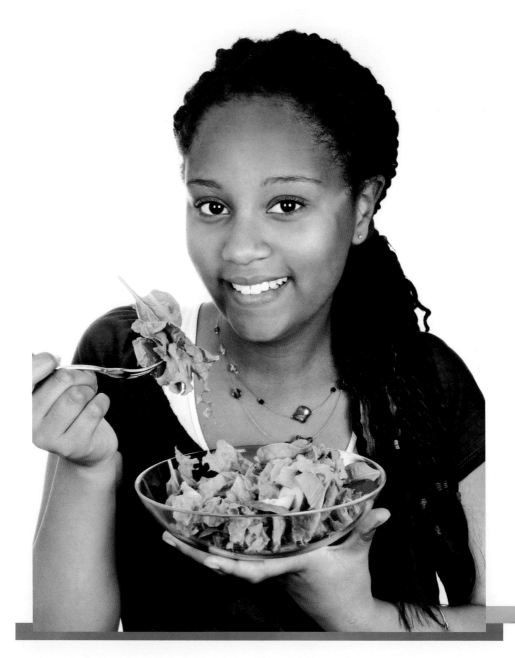

Eating a healthy diet high in vitamins and minerals and low in fat helps keep a person's body in the best shape to deal with the rigors of treatment and to heal.

Supplements and Nutrition

People take herbal supplements for a variety of reasons. The effects of chemicals extracted (removed) from plants include relaxing the body, helping one get to sleep, improving immune system functioning, treating constipation and diarrhea, and improving one's mood, among others. Even though they occur naturally, these plant extracts are still chemicals. Therefore, they can have side effects, just like man-made medicines. If you are thinking of taking an herbal supplement, talk to your doctor first, especially when you are taking hormone replacement medication. The active ingredient in an herbal supplement may interact with the medication that your doctor prescribes.

Proper nutrition is critical to keeping the body healthy so that it can heal properly. Even when stressed out by a disease or treatment, it is important to eat regularly and eat a well-balanced diet. It is essential to eat regularly, even if stress is affecting one's appetite. A diet high in fruits, vegetables, whole grains, and protein and low in fat can help keep the immune system and body strong and better able to cope with treatment and recovery.

TEN GREAT QUESTIONS
TO ASK YOUR DOCTOR

1. What kind of thyroid cancer do I have?

2. What is the prognosis?

3. What types of treatment might work? What are their pros and cons?

4. Whom could I see for a second opinion?

5. How much experience do you have treating this type of cancer?

6. How soon do I need to make a decision about treatment?

7. Do you have information on support groups for people with thyroid cancer?

8. How long will it take for me to recover from treatment?

9. Will I need to take medication after treatment? What kind?

10. What will I have to do after treatment to stay healthy?

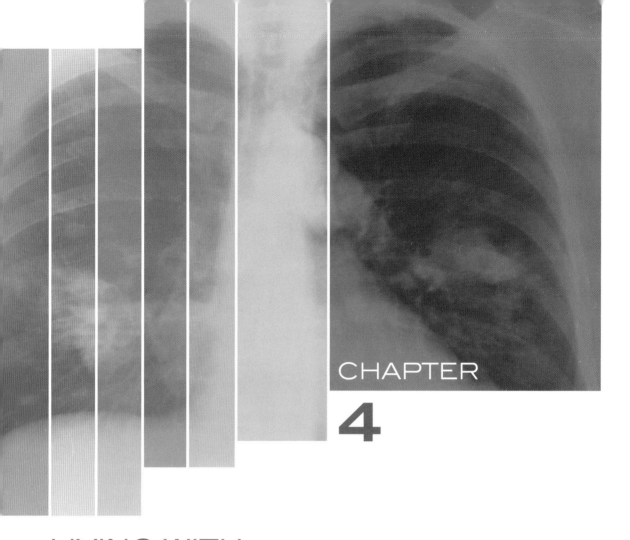

LIVING WITH THYROID CANCER

Being diagnosed with cancer causes immense stress and anxiety about many issues. People rarely die of thyroid cancer, but there are a number of other serious concerns. Those who are diagnosed with thyroid cancer are usually faced with having surgery. Because this surgery is going to be done at a visible point on the front of the neck, many people are concerned about how the procedure will affect their appearance.

A second fear is that the cancer will come back or spread to other organs in the future, causing health problems. Patients may also have concerns about the effects on their body from the loss of the thyroid

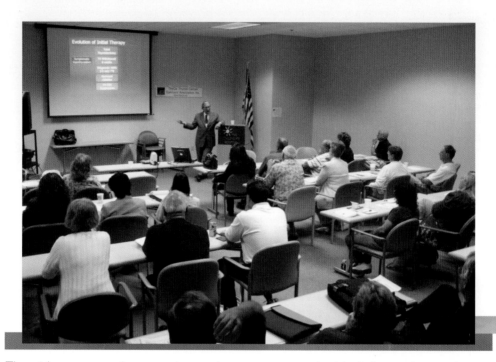

Thyroid cancer patients and caregivers can get valuable information and advice by attending educational events sponsored by organizations such as the American Thyroid Association.

hormones produced by the thyroid gland or about side effects that can result from hormone replacement therapy. In addition, treatment is often physically and mentally stressful. The side effects of treatment may make one feel sick and fatigued. The mere fact of having cancer often affects how people feel about themselves and life in general. Therefore, having support at this difficult time can be very important.

Some people find it valuable to talk to a mental health professional or counselor. The best choice may be a professional who works regularly with cancer patients and their families. Hospitals and oncologists (doctors who specialize in cancer treatment) can often recommend therapists who have expertise in this area.

CANCER SUPPORT GROUPS

Support groups can be joined in person or over the Internet. The following are some organizations that offer lists of local support groups and/or online support groups:

—— American Cancer Society: www.cancer.org
—— American Thyroid Association: www.thyroid.org
—— Cancer Care: www.supportgroups.cancercare.org
—— Daily Strength, Thyroid Cancer Support Group: www. dailystrength.org/c/Thyroid-Cancer/support-group
—— ThyCa: Thyroid Cancer Survivors Association: www.thyca.org
—— The Wellness Community: www.thewellnesscommunity.org

Moreover, patients should check with the facility where they obtain treatment, since the facility may also sponsor cancer support groups or keep a list of local community groups.

There are various types of support groups for people who are being treated for cancer and their families. In addition to providing emotional support while going through treatment, the members of such groups may also be able to provide advice on how to deal with the effects of treatment.

REPLACING THYROID HORMONES

Once the thyroid is removed, the body has no way of producing thyroid hormone, which is critical to healthy mental and physical functioning. Therefore, a person who has a thyroidectomy must replace the thyroid hormone. To do that, he or she takes a synthetic (man-made) form of

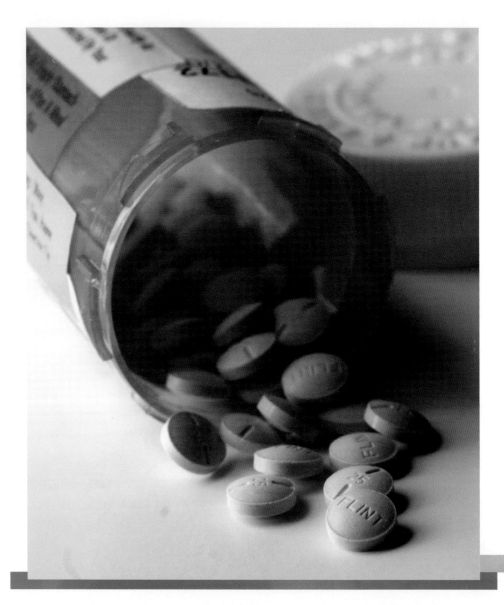

Synthetic hormones such as Synthroid, seen here as a prescribed tablet, have made it possible for people who have had their thyroid gland removed to maintain a normal metabolism.

thyroid hormone T4, called levothyroxine, in pill form. Two commonly prescribed versions of synthetic thyroid hormone are Synthroid by Abbott Laboratories and Levothroid by Forest Pharmaceuticals.

Aside from keeping the body properly regulated, maintaining an adequate level of thyroid hormone helps control the amount of thyroid-stimulating hormone (TSH). Too much TSH can stimulate the growth of cells, including any cancer cells remaining in the body. Consequently, keeping the level from getting too high is beneficial. When a person takes a synthetic thyroid hormone, his or her doctor will periodically schedule blood tests to verify that the correct level of thyroid hormone is present in the blood so that the person doesn't develop symptoms of hyperthyroidism or hypothyroidism.

Recovery and Follow-Up

After treatment for thyroid cancer, the doctor continues to monitor the patient, checking at regular intervals to make sure that the cancer does not recur. This can happen if cells had already split off from the tumor and invaded other organs before the thyroid cancer was treated. Doctors may use thyroid imaging and blood tests to verify that a patient is still cancer-free. When thyroid cancer does recur, it often appears in the lymph nodes, lungs, bones, or remnants of thyroid tissue not completely removed during surgery. Even when thyroid cancer recurs, it can be treated successfully in many instances.

Long-Term Effects of Thyroid Gland Removal

In patients with low-risk papillary and follicular cancer, thyroid hormones are typically retained at near-normal levels through thyroid medication. In these cases, there are usually no serious long-term effects of thyroid removal, as long as thyroid levels are monitored regularly by blood tests

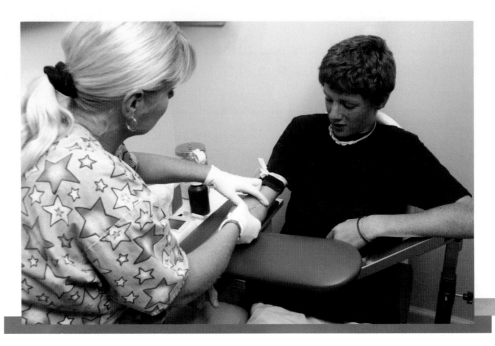

People taking replacement hormones need to have simple blood tests performed periodically to verify that the amount of hormones in their blood remains at the optimum level.

to verify that the proper dose of medication is taken. If the level of thyroid hormones becomes too low, the person may experience the effects of hypothyroidism, including fatigue, weight gain, and depression. It is important that a person who experiences such symptoms contact his or her doctor to test the level of thyroid hormones in the blood. The most common blood test for thyroid levels determines the amount of TSH and T4 circulating in the blood. These tests can be a little tricky to interpret due to the normal feedback mechanisms, though. For example, if a person has symptoms of hypothyroidism but the TSH level is normal, the doctor will also test for free T4 and T3 to directly measure the amount of these hormones in the blood.

Coping with Cancer in the Family

When someone in the family becomes seriously ill, this can put great stress on family relationships, especially if cancer is involved. If the person involved is a parent, children in the family are likely not only to worry about the sick parent, but also fear what will happen if their parent should die. This is natural because young people rely on their parents for emotional and practical support. The good news about thyroid cancer is that it is usually not fatal. However, a sick parent may still be less able to give attention to his or her children. This can make children feel angry and resentful. At the same time, they may feel self-conscious about their feelings. It is normal to have these kinds of feelings. If possible, it is a good idea to talk to other people—friends, a counselor, or members of a local or online support group.

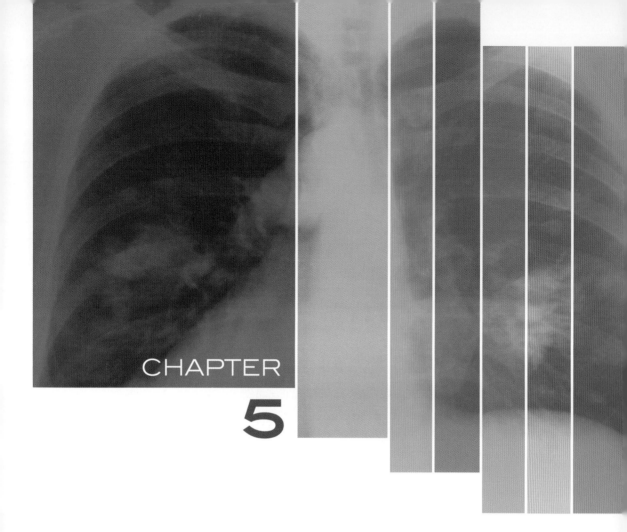

CHAPTER

5

THE FUTURE

Advances in technology have provided new tools to solve the problem of treating cancer. Doctors have a greater knowledge of genetics than ever before, and new tools such as lasers and advanced forms of medical imaging may someday allow for better treatment.

RESEARCH INTO NEW DIAGNOSTIC TECHNIQUES

Most of the research into new diagnostic techniques is aimed at improving existing techniques by applying new technologies. An example of this

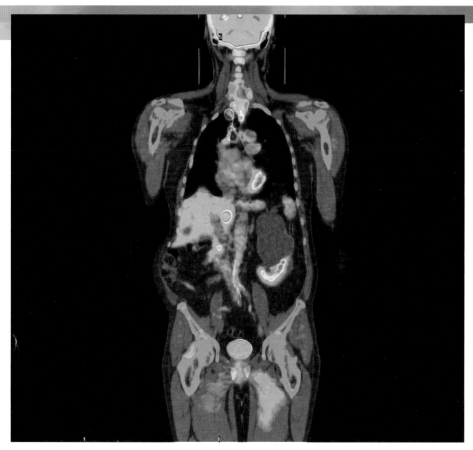

This positron emission tomography (PET) scan shows where thyroid cancer cells have spread. They're visible in the patient's liver, colon, and lung.

practice is a study being undertaken using positron emission tomography (PET) scanning. PET scans are one means of imaging used to detect thyroid cancer cells that may have spread. PET scans for thyroid cancer are done using sugar that has been combined with radioactive atoms. The sugar is readily taken up by cancer cells because they are growing rapidly; iodine is commonly taken up by thyroid cells. A detector scans the patient's body, and the areas with various levels of radioactive activity show up in different colors, allowing doctors to detect the presence of cells that might be cancerous. A study is being undertaken to establish if administering a genetically engineered form of TSH prior to scanning provides more sensitive detection of cancer cells than conventional PET scanning.

Another approach to improved diagnosis being tested is the use of gene profiling to differentiate between benign and cancerous cells after biopsy. The question being explored is if DNA analysis would provide a more accurate means of identifying whether or not cells in the sample are cancerous than current methods.

RESEARCH INTO NEW TREATMENTS

Clinical trials are under way to explore a number of ways to improve the treatment of thyroid cancer. One study, led by the U.S. National Institute of Diabetes and Digestive and Kidney Diseases, is aimed at reducing potential side effects from radioactive iodine treatment. Most papillary and follicular cancers can be successfully treated by thyroid removal, followed by treatment with radioactive iodine. However, there is concern about the long-term effects of exposure to the radiation in radioactive iodine. Therefore, one study is examining whether or not giving patients lithium carbonate during treatment would enhance the uptake of iodine by cancerous thyroid cells. If so, lower doses of radioactive iodine could be used for treatment, reducing the risk of future problems from exposure to radiation.

One of the problems in treating thyroid cancer is the poor response of medullary thyroid cancer to radioactive iodine therapy. An approach being researched is making types of thyroid cancer that are not easily treated with radioactive iodine more sensitive to the compound. The U.S. National Cancer Institute is leading a study to explore whether or not the compound valproic acid can be used to make

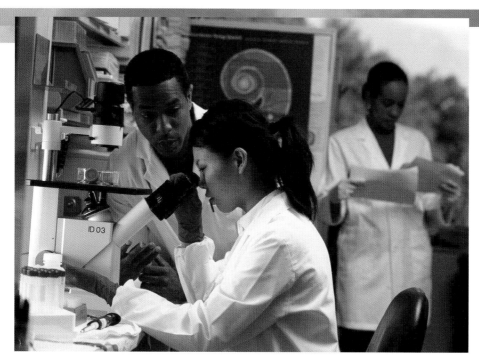

Researchers around the world, supported by government agencies and private pharmaceutical companies, are studying ways to stop cancer cells from forming and destroy them when they occur.

thyroid cancers that don't respond to radioactive iodine treatment more sensitive to it.

A second approach is to find alternatives to radioactive iodine treatment for use in those types of thyroid cancer that don't respond to it. The National Cancer Institute is sponsoring a study using the medication sorafenib to see if blocking the enzymes necessary for cell growth and blocking the blood flow to the tumor can successfully treat thyroid cancer. In another experimental study sponsored by the National Cancer Institute, the medication bortezomib is being tested to see if blocking the proteins needed for cell growth can treat metastatic thyroid cancer. The National Cancer Institute is also supporting a study of vandetanib, another blocker of critical proteins within cells, to treat medullary thyroid cancer in young patients.

Growing extra blood vessels to feed tumors created by fast-growing cells is critical to cancer cells' survival. In a study being funded in France by the pharmaceutical company Pfizer, researchers are seeing whether or not the drug sunitinib would sufficiently interfere with the ability of tumors to generate blood vessels. If so, this could result in choking off the tumors' blood supply and providing another means to treat thyroid cancer. Another trial involving blocking tumors' blood supply is being carried out at the University Hospital in Lund, Sweden. This study is aimed at treating anaplastic thyroid cancer and uses a combination of the drugs bevacizumab and doxorubicin after thyroid removal to treat residual and metastasized thyroid cancer cells. Similar medications are being experimented with to treat other types of solid tumors as well.

Research into New Surgical Treatments

Another area being explored is improved methods of thyroid surgery. One approach involves the use of lasers, rather than scalpels, to perform thyroid surgery. Surgical lasers produce a precise beam of intense light that can be used to destroy carefully targeted tissue in the body. The laser is inserted through an endoscope, a narrow tube passed down the patient's throat. BioTex, Inc., and Rhode Island Hospital are one research team currently investigating the use of lasers to treat benign thyroid nodules. The advantages of using laser surgery are that it can very precisely target nodules without damaging the surrounding tissue, it causes less bleeding, and it has less chance of infection than making an open cut with a scalpel. The disadvantages are that it is very expensive and that nodules may recur, so treatment might have to be repeated.

CLINICAL TRIALS

Many of the new approaches to the diagnosis and treatment of thyroid cancer discussed in this chapter are currently being explored through clinical trials. A clinical trial is used to see if a proposed treatment works and is safe enough to use in medical practice. These treatments have to first demonstrate enough usefulness and safety in laboratory and animal tests to be tried in people. In the United States, clinical trials are overseen by government agencies such as the National Institutes of Health and the Food and Drug Administration. In Canada, they are overseen by Health Canada.

The treatments being used in clinical trials have not yet been proved effective and safe in people, so there are significant risks. However, if conventional therapy is not successful in treating a person's thyroid cancer, he or she may choose to join a clinical trial.

There are many risks in undergoing an experimental treatment. The treatment may have side effects, which your doctor should fully discuss with you. In addition, there is no guarantee that it will work. However, people who have a form of thyroid cancer that doesn't respond to other treatments may feel that the possibility that the treatment will work is worth the risk. Also, some people feel that even if it doesn't help them, volunteering to try it will help advance scientists' knowledge and may improve the chances of finding a treatment that does help someone else.

Information on clinical trials for the treatment of thyroid cancer can be obtained from the U.S. National Institutes of Health clinical trials Web site at http://clinicaltrials.gov.

In a different approach, Johnson & Johnson and the Brazil Society of Head and Neck Surgery are working to see if Johnson & Johnson's Harmonic Scalpel is a better tool than a conventional scalpel for performing surgery on benign and malignant thyroid tumors. The Harmonic Scalpel uses an electrical current to generate a vibration. It cuts via vibration and, at the same time, causes the blood in the wound to coagulate (thicken) to stop bleeding. It can do this because the vibration alters the proteins in much the same way that whipping egg white causes it to thicken. Researchers are looking at elements such as outcome, recovery time, and improvement in side effects from surgery, among other factors.

Gene Therapy for Thyroid Cancer

"Genetic engineering" is a term that means changing genes so that they perform specific functions. Over the past twenty-five years, scientists have developed many technological tools and techniques that allow them to alter genes. This therapy genetically engineers techniques to treat disease. Gene therapies are still mostly experimental, and those for thyroid cancer are in the clinical trials phase, in which researchers are attempting to establish if they are effective and safe. Scientists throughout the world are exploring gene therapy–based solutions to various types of cancer, including thyroid cancer.

Gene therapy for thyroid cancer is primarily aimed at treating medullary and anaplastic thyroid cancers because they don't respond well to radioactive iodine treatment. The idea behind gene therapy for thyroid cancer is that if one could insert a gene into thyroid cancer cells that makes them susceptible to a medication or chemical compound, the patient could then be given that compound to kill the cancer cells. In Europe and China, studies are being conducted using various antibiotics as the compound used to kill thyroid cancer cells that have been treated with gene therapy to make them susceptible.

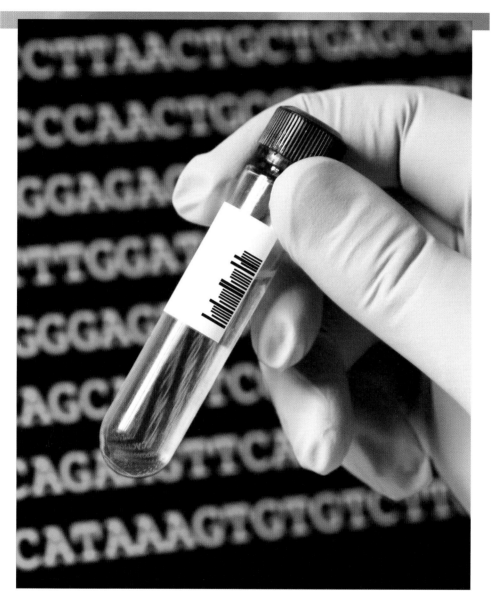

Throughout the world, scientists are working on research into gene-based solutions to disease, such as thyroid cancer. They use techniques such as gene sequencing to understand the genes that are involved.

The basis for gene therapy is as follows: if one can put a new gene into an existing cell, that gene will be copied into the new cells as they reproduce. They will then have whatever characteristic the new gene gives—in this case, susceptibility to medication.

To insert the gene into the cell, it is necessary to penetrate the wall surrounding the nucleus to reach the chromosomes that contain the genes. Viruses are able to penetrate the membrane, which they do to inject their own DNA to infect the cell. Therefore, viruses make an excellent delivery mechanism for new genes. Before scientists can use viruses for gene delivery, they must make sure that the virus is rendered harmless so that it can't cause infection. Then the scientists attach the gene they want to deliver to the virus. To make sure that noncancerous cells are not killed, the gene that is inserted is a gene that normally exists in thyroid cells, only altered so that it is sensitive to the compound in question. Next, the viruses are placed in a solution that is given to the patient intravenously (through a vein). The viruses travel through the patient's bloodstream and infect thyroid cells wherever they have spread in the body. As the cancer cells reproduce, the new gene is copied with the other genes. The patient is then given the antibiotic to which the gene makes the cell sensitive, and the cells are killed.

This chapter has examined some of the new approaches to the diagnosis and treatment of thyroid cancer. Continuing advances in technology make it likely that new methods of diagnosis and treatment for this cancer will continue to be developed, offering hope to those who currently have forms of thyroid cancer that are difficult to treat with conventional therapies.

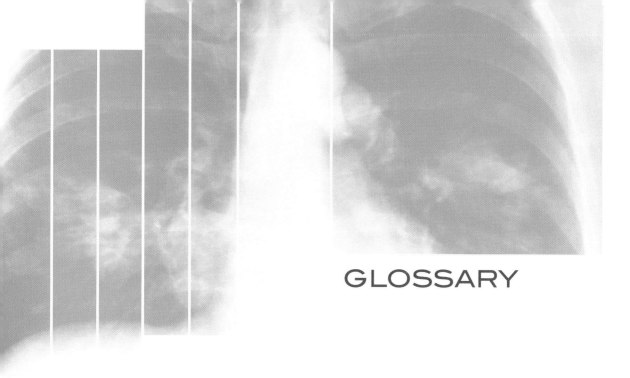

GLOSSARY

beneficial Good for one.

benign Noncancerous.

colloid Fluid that is produced in the thyroid and includes the iodine-containing protein thyroglobulin.

consume To eat.

differentiated Developed into a recognizable cell.

epithelial cell A cell that lines or covers a gland or organ.

esophagus The tube in the throat that food goes down on its way to the stomach.

extract To remove from.

follicle A spherical pouch in an organ or gland.

goiter An enlarged or swollen thyroid gland.

hormone A chemical produced in the body that affects the functioning of the body.

incidence The occurrence, rate, or frequency of a disease.

incision A cut made during surgery.

intravenous Through a vein.

lymph node Glandlike tissue in the neck that stores immune system cells for fighting infection.

malignant A type of cancer that spreads.

metastasis The spreading of cancer from the point of origin to other organs.

nodule A lump made up of cells that may be malignant or benign.

oncogene A gene that can cause a cell to become cancerous.

optimal At the best level.

parathyroid glands Small glands located behind the thyroid gland that control the usage of calcium in the body.

pituitary gland A gland located at the back of the brain.

receptor A socketlike projection on the wall of a cell to which chemicals such as hormones attach.

secrete To generate or put out.

sporadic Occurring occasionally and unpredictably.

synthetic Man-made.

thyroidectomy The surgical removal of the thyroid gland.

trachea Windpipe.

undifferentiated Not having the characteristics of an identifiable type of cell.

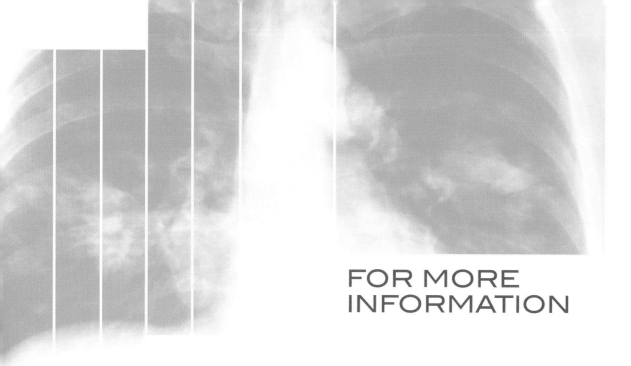

FOR MORE
INFORMATION

American Cancer Society
1599 Clifton Road NE
Atlanta, GA 30329
(800) ACS-2345 [227-2345]
Web site: http://www.cancer.org
The American Cancer Society provides resources including publications, an informative Web site, and assistance by phone.

American Institute of Cancer Research
1759 R Street NW
Washington, DC 20009
(202) 328-7226
Web site: http://www.aicr.org
This organization provides the latest information on cancer
   research activities and a variety of printed resources on cancer.

American Thyroid Association
6066 Leesburg Pike, Suite 550

Falls Church, VA 22041
(703) 998-8890
Web site: http://www.thyroid.org
This organization provides news, information, and publications, including publications for patients.

Canadian Cancer Society
10 Alcorn Avenue, Suite 2000
Toronto, ON M4V 3B1
Canada
(416) 961-7223
Web site: http://www.cancer.ca
This organization provides the latest news on cancer in Canada and
  information on specific types of cancer.

Kids Konnected
27071 Cabot Road, Suite 102
Laguna, CA 92653
(949) 582-5443
Web site: http://wwwkidskonnected.org
This organization, supported by many major corporations, is devoted
  to supporting kids who have a parent with cancer or have lost a
  parent to it. It has separate resources for children and teenagers,
  including camps, support groups, a Web site, and more.

National Cancer Institute
6116 Executive Boulevard
Bethesda, MD 20892-8322
(800) 422-6237
Web site: http://www.cancer.gov

Part of the U.S. National Institutes of Health, this institute provides
information on thyroid cancer, including information on clinical trials
currently recruiting patients.

National Coalition for Cancer Survivorship
1010 Wayne Avenue, Suite 770
Silver Spring, MD 20910
(301) 650-9127/(888) 650-9127
Web site: http://www.canceradvocacy.org
This is the oldest survivor-led cancer advocacy organization in the
country. Its members advocate for high-quality cancer care for all
Americans and seek to empower cancer survivors. The organization
also provides patient education about cancer.

Thyroid Foundation of Canada
1669 Jalna Boulevard, Suite 803
London, ON N6E 3S1
Canada
(519) 649-5478/(800) 267-8822 (in Canada)
Web site: http://www.thyroid.ca
This organization provides publications on thyroid health and disorders, including nodules and cancer, as well as public lectures related
to thyroid health.

WEB SITES

Due to the changing nature of Internet links, Rosen Publishing has
developed an online list of Web sites related to the subject of this book.
This site is updated regularly. Please use this link to access the list:

http://www.rosenlinks.com/cms/thyr

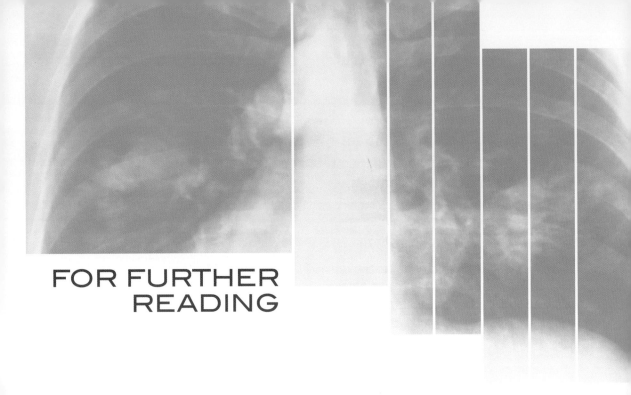

FOR FURTHER READING

American Cancer Society. *QuickFacts Thyroid Cancer*. Atlanta, GA: American Cancer Society, 2009.

Burch, Warner M. *100 Questions and Answers About Thyroid Disorders*. Sudbury, MA: Jones & Bartlett, 2008.

Caldwell, Wilma A., ed. *Cancer Information for Teens: Health Tips About Cancer Awareness, Prevention, Diagnosis, and Treatment*. Detroit, MI: Omnigraphics, 2004.

Cefrey, Holly. *Coping with Cancer*. New York, NY: Rosen Publishing Group, 2003.

Daniels, Gilbert H., and Colin M. Dayan. *Fast Facts: Thyroid Disorders*. Oxford, England: Health Press, 2006.

Dreyer, ZoAnn. *Teen Guides: Living with Cancer*. New York, NY: Checkmark Books, 2008.

Greenstein, Ben. *The Endocrine System at a Glance*. Malden, MA: Blackwell, 2006.

Klosterman, Lorrie. *The Endocrine System*. Tarrytown, NY: Marshall Cavendish, 2008.

Lew, Kristi. *The Truth About Cancer: Understanding and Fighting a Deadly Disease*. Berkeley Heights, NJ: Enslow, 2009.

Mooney, Belinda. *Cancer*. Chicago, IL: Greenhaven Press, 2007.

Nelson, Sheila. *Youth with Cancer: Facing the Shadows*. Broomall, PA: Mason Crest, 2007.

Rubin, Alan. *Thyroid for Dummies*. Hoboken, NJ: Wiley, 2006.

Rushton, Lynette. *The Endocrine System*. New York, NY: Chelsea House, 2009.

Shepard, Glenda. *Thyroid Cancer for Beginners*. Central Milton Keynes, England: AuthorHouse, 2009.

Silverthorne, Elizabeth. *Cancer*. San Diego, CA: Lucent Books, 2009.

Therrien, Patricia. *An Enemy Within: Overcoming Cancer and Other Life-Threatening Diseases*. Broomall, PA: Mason Crest, 2008.

Van Nostrand, D., G. Bloom, and L. Wartofsky. *Thyroid Cancer: A Guide for Patients*. Pasadena, MD: Keystone Press, 2004.

Wyborny, Sheila. *Cancer Treatments*. Chicago, IL: Blackbirch, 2005.

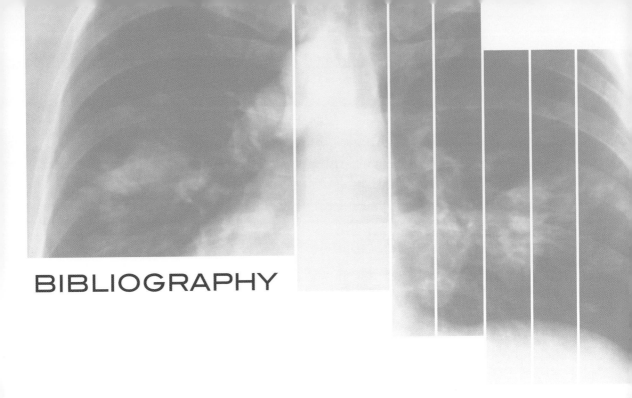

BIBLIOGRAPHY

American Cancer Society. "Detailed Guide: Thyroid Cancer."
    Retrieved January 24, 2010 (http://www.cancer.org/docroot/
    cri/content/cri_2_4_1x_what_are_the_key_statistics_for_
    thyroid_cancer_43.asp).

American Society of Clinical Oncology. "Thyroid Cancer."
    Retrieved January 22, 2010 (http://www.cancer.net/patient/
    Cancer+Types/Thyroid+Cancer).

American Thyroid Association. "Thyroid Cancer FAQs." Retrieved
    January 22, 2010 (http://www.thyroid.org/patients/faqs/cancer_
    of_thyroid.html).

Cancer.net. "Thyroid Cancer." Retrieved January 30, 2010
    (http://www.cancer.net/patient/Cancer+Types/Thyroid+
    Cancer?sectionTitle=Clinical Trials Resources).

Columbia University Department of Otolaryngology Head
    and Neck Surgery. "Transnasal Flexible Laryngoscopy (TFL)."
    Retrieved January 29, 2010 (http://www.entcolumbia.org/tfl.html).

Friedman, Theodore C., and Winnie Yu. *The Everything Health
    Guide to Thyroid Disease.* Avon, MA: F & W Media, 2007.

Mahoney, Martin C., Silvana Lawvere, Karen L. Falkner, Yuri I. Averkin, Vladislav A. Ostapenko, Arthur M. Michalek, Kirsten B. Moysich, and Philip L. McCarthy. "Thyroid Cancer Incidence Trends in Belarus: Examining the Impact of Chernobyl." *International Journal of Epidemiology,* Vol. 33, pp. 1–9, 2004. Retrieved January 27, 2010 (http://ije.oxfordjournals.org/cgi/reprint/dyh201v1.pdf).

Mayo Clinic. "Thyroid Cancer." Retrieved February 2, 2010 (http://www.mayoclinic.com/print/thyroid-cancer/DS00492/DSECTION=all&METHOD=print).

Medline Plus. "Thyroid Cancer." National Institutes of Health. Retrieved February 2, 2010 (http://www.nlm.nih.gov/medlineplus/thyroidcancer.html).

Memorial Sloan-Kettering Cancer Center. "Thyroid Cancer." Retrieved January 30, 2010 (http://www.mskcc.org/mskcc/html/447.cfm).

National Cancer Institute. "Fact Sheet: Detection." Retrieved January 28, 2010 (http://www.cancer.gov/cancertopics/factsheet/Detection/staging).

Rosenthal, Sara. *The Thyroid Sourcebook.* 5th ed. New York, NY: McGraw-Hill, 2008.

Skugor, Mario, and Jesse Bryant Wilder. *The Cleveland Clinic Guide to Thyroid Disorders.* New York, NY: Kaplan Publishing, 2009.

Thyroid Cancer Survivors Association. "Thyroid Cancer Facts." Retrieved January 30, 2010 (http://www.thyca.org/thyroidcancerfacts.htm).

Thyroid Foundation of Canada. "Thyroid Cancer." Retrieved January 30, 2010 (http://www.thyroid.ca/Guides/HG12.html).

University of Pennsylvania Abramson Cancer Center. "Thyroid Cancer: The Basics." Retrieved January 30, 2010 (http://www.oncolink.org/types/article.cfm?c=20&s=65&ss=513&id=107&CFID=25494828&CFTOKEN=18182455).

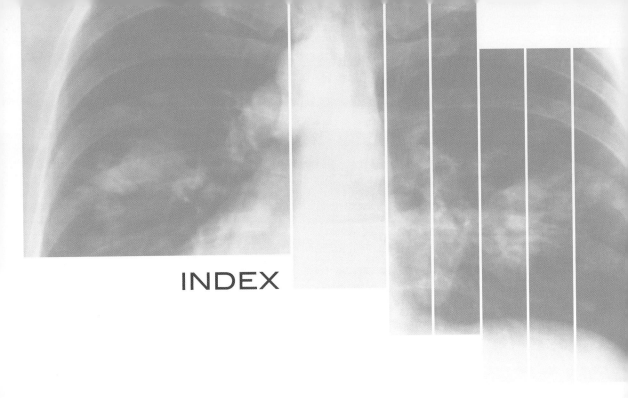

INDEX

ABOUT THE AUTHOR

Jeri Freedman earned a B.A. degree from Harvard University. For fifteen years, she worked for companies in the medical field. Among the numerous books she has written for young adults are *Hemophilia*, *Hepatitis B*, *Lymphoma: Current and Emerging Trends in Detection and Treatment*, *How Do We Know About Genetics and Heredity?*, *The Mental and Physical Effects of Obesity*, *Autism*, *Tay-Sachs Disease*, and *Ovarian Cancer*.

PHOTO CREDITS

Cover, pp. 1, 17 Science Photo Library/Custom Medical Stock Photo; pp. 3, 7, 14, 25, 37, 44, 53, 55, 58, 60, 62, back cover National Cancer Institute; pp. 4–5 (bottom) LifeART image © 2010 Lippincott Williams & Wilkins. All rights reserved; pp. 5 (top), 38 Thyroid Cancers Survivors Association; p. 8 © De Agostini Picture Library/De Agostini/Getty Images; p. 10 National Institutes of Health; pp. 12, 19 Dr. Gladden Willis/Visuals Unlimited; pp. 15, 47 National Cancer Institute; pp. 20–21 Radiation Protection Division/Health Protection Agency/Photo Researchers; p. 27 National Medical Slide Bank/Custom Medical Stock Photo; p. 30 © Mark Harmel/Stone/Getty Images; p. 34 Shutterstock; p. 40 © Tony Cenicola/The New York Times/Redux Pictures; p. 42 istockphoto/Thinkstock; p. 45 © ISM/Phototake; p. 51 © www.istockphoto.com/dra_schwartz.

Designer: Evelyn Horovicz; Editor: Kathy Kuhtz Campbell;
Photo Researcher: Marty Levick